I0065635

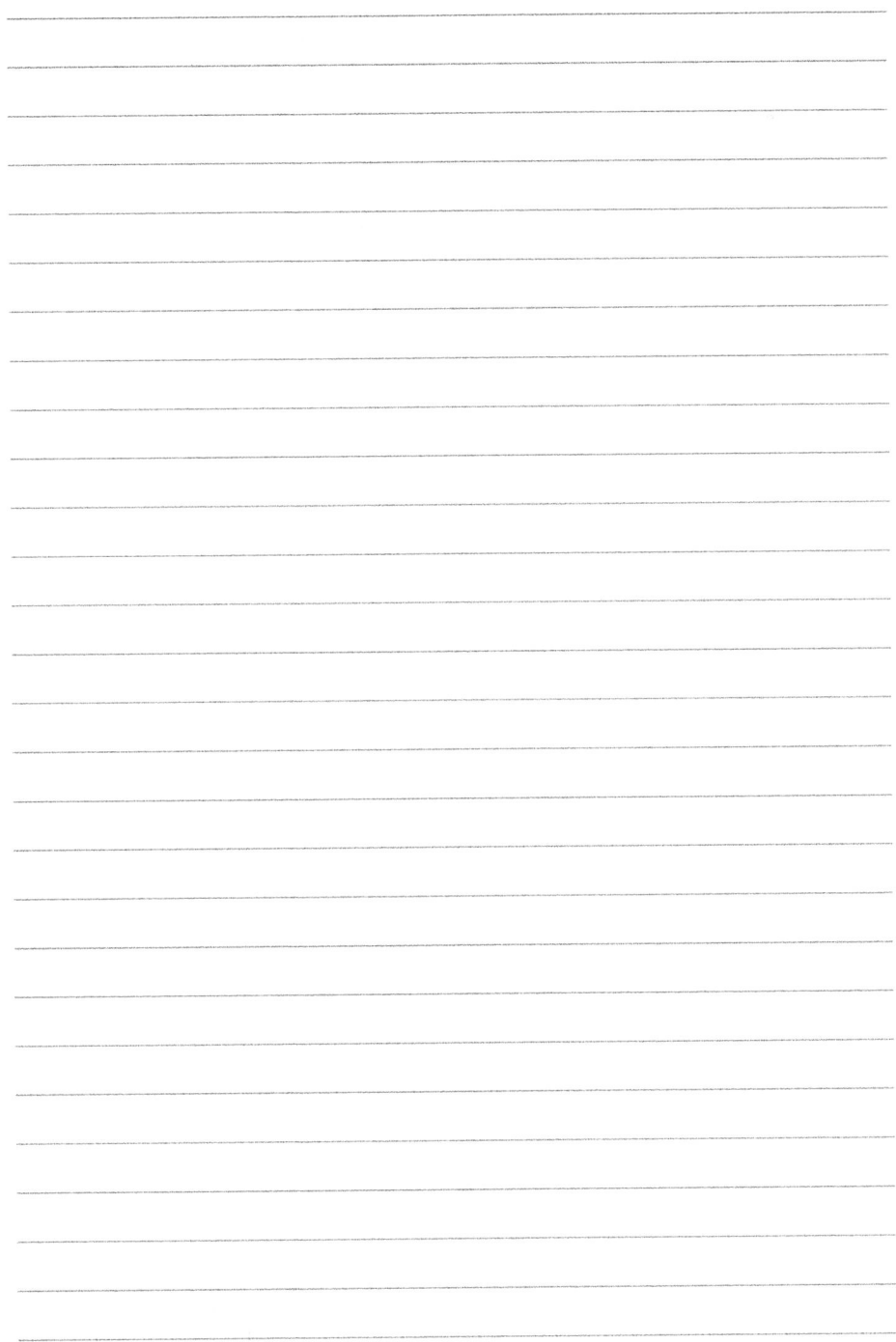

First Responder Paramedic Journal Notebook
Greatest Teams In The World First Responder Journal Series
EMS Gift Book For Paramedics and EMT Professionals
Paperback ISBN: 978-1-989733-43-1
Copyright Dunhill Clare Publishing 2020
All Rights Reserved. Cover Design by Sharon Purtill

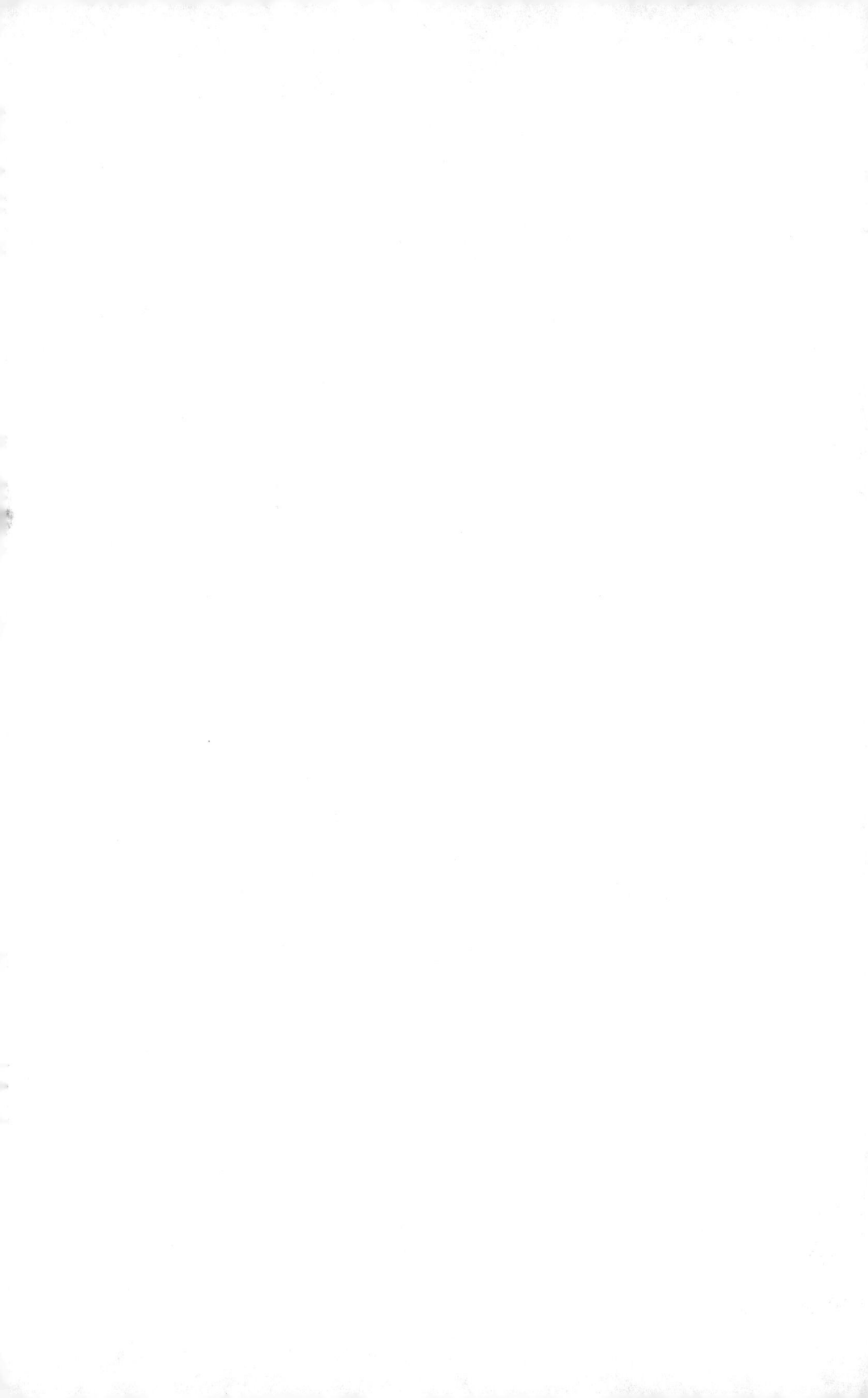

www.ingramcontent.com/pod-product-compliance
Lightning Source LLC
Chambersburg PA
CBHW071431210326
41597CB00020B/3745